David, We're PREGNANT!

101 cartoons for
Expecting Parents
by Lynn Johnston

MEADOWBROOK PRESS
18318 Minnetonka Blvd.
Deephaven, Minnesota 55391

Meadowbrook Press Edition
10th Printing February 1982

PRINTED IN THE UNITED STATES OF AMERICA

Library of Congress Catalog Number: 77-82214

ISBN 0-915658-04-6

Once upon a time there were no cartoons on the ceiling of my examining room.

From my point of view, of course, the examining room was always an interesting place where I met fascinating people, with perplexing problems for me to solve. The relationship was simple and direct. The patients had questions. I had gone to medical school and learned answers. The examining room was the place where the questions and the answers got together. Both patient and doctor went in for the same purpose, and both went out satisfied.

One day a perceptive woman, who had lain all too long on the table counting the dots on an otherwise blank ceiling, asked me why I didn't put any pictures up there. I didn't have a good answer, but I realized it was a good question. And I was struck with the realization that the patient's point of view from the examining table was very different from the doctor's point of view. A host of new questions started to crowd in.

When does pregnancy really begin? Is it, like we were taught in school, at the precise moment when sperm and egg join together, or is it earlier, when a couple start to plan and yearn for a family? Or is it perhaps later, with the realization of pregnancy, and the growing awareness of the life within?

What is pregnancy? Is it the weight gains and the blood pressures and the morning sicknesses and the strange symptoms the doctor sees? Or is it the hopes and fears, and joys and tremblings, and a new body to adjust to, and a new shape to learn to love? Is it a time for parents to prepare for their new exciting role to come?

What are prenatal classes? A passing fad to keep patients occupied? Or an opportunity for us to learn about our bodies and ourselves, to learn the skills needed for the awesome task ahead?

What is labor? Is it a series of uterine contractions working to dilate the cervix and expel a new baby into the world? Or is it a dreaded yet anticipated experience, unknown and unknowable, through which one must pass with only old wives' tales and untested prenatal classes as uncertain guides?

Indeed, what is the new baby? A little patient to be weighed and tested, and formulas to be adjusted? Or a new individual who will change lovers into parents, and mates into a family, with new joys and sleepless nights?

There are many books about pregnancy, but most are written from the professional's point of view. The patient's answers to these questions are rarely expressed. In this book, Lynn has given the parents' viewpoint, clearly and pointedly. For parents, for parents-to-be, and for professionals too.

And now I have cartoons on my ceiling.

MURRAY W. ENKIN, M.D.

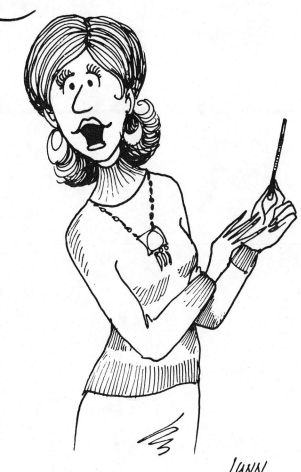

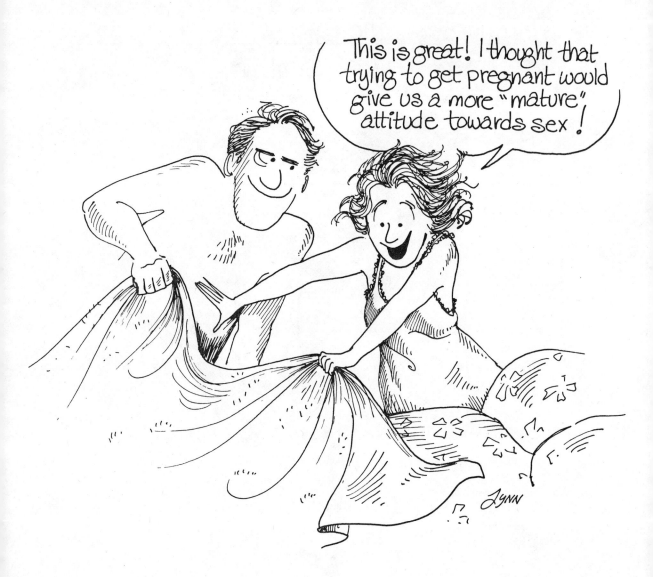

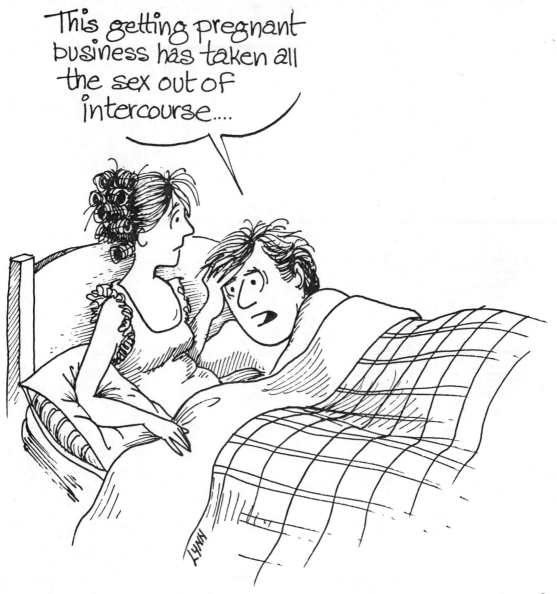

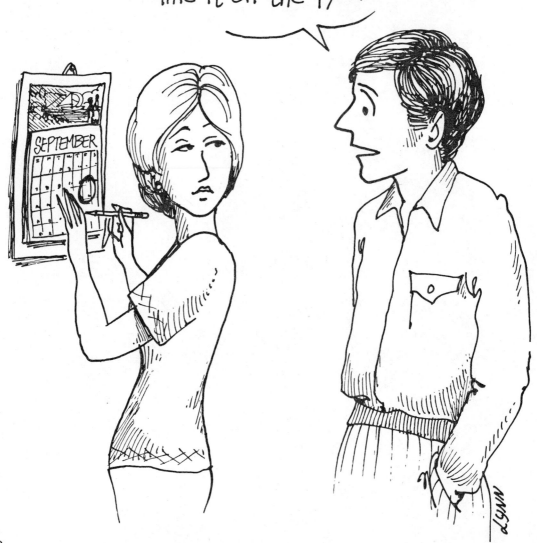

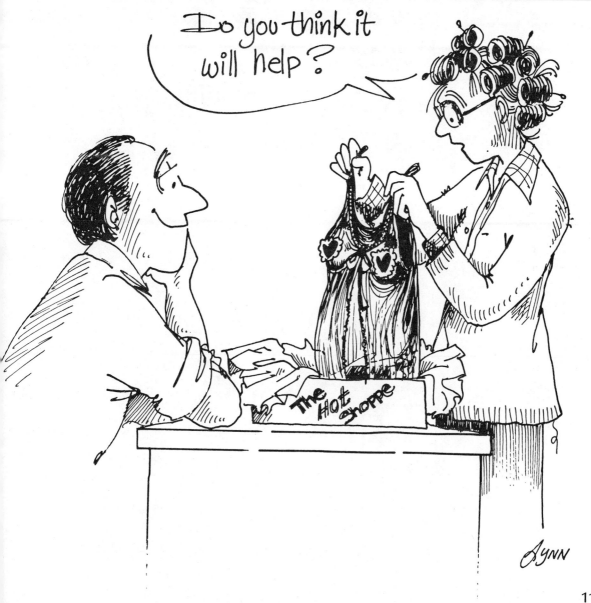

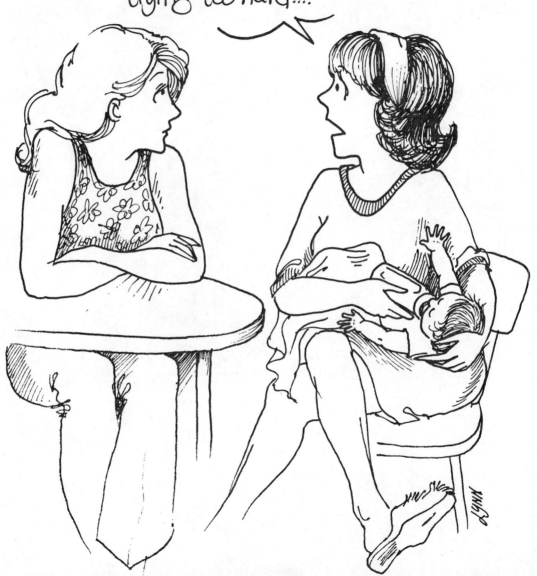

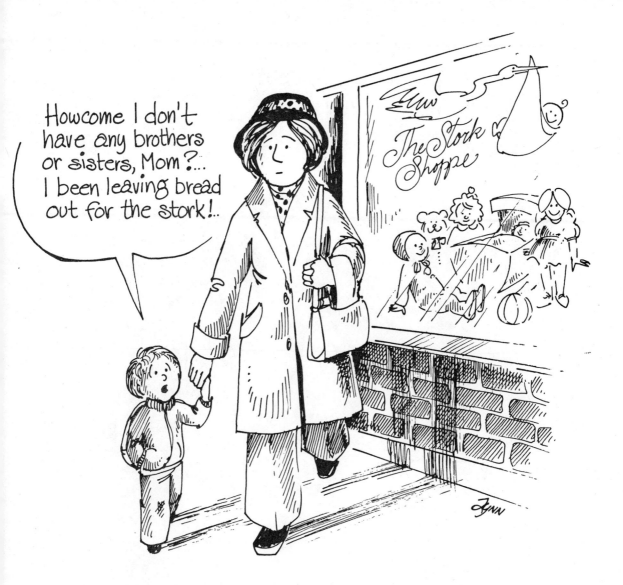

13

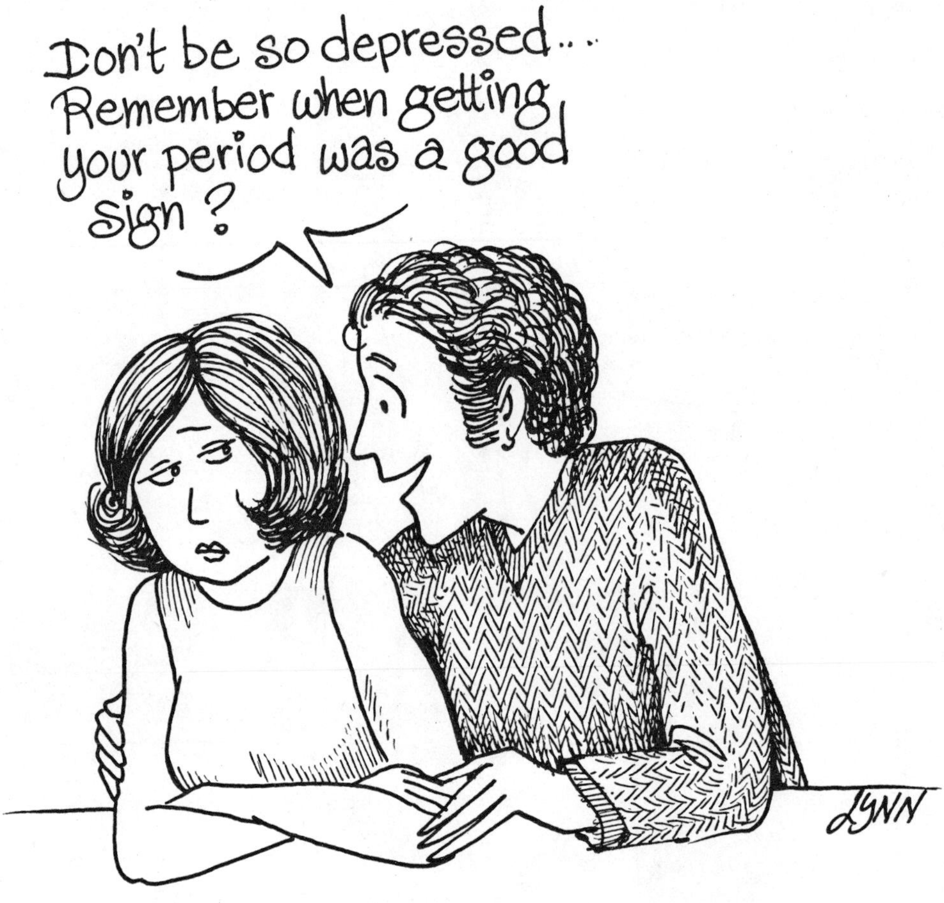
Don't be so depressed....
Remember when getting
your period was a good
sign ?
LYNN

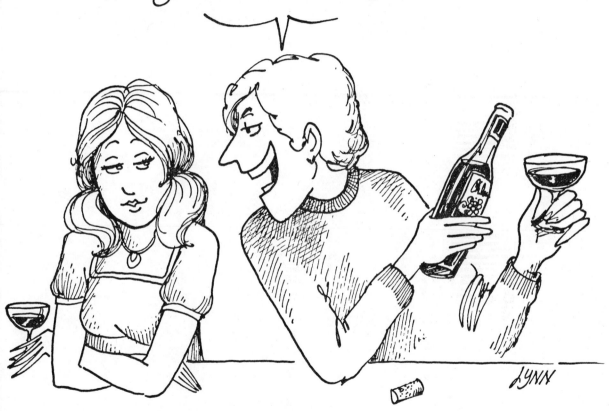

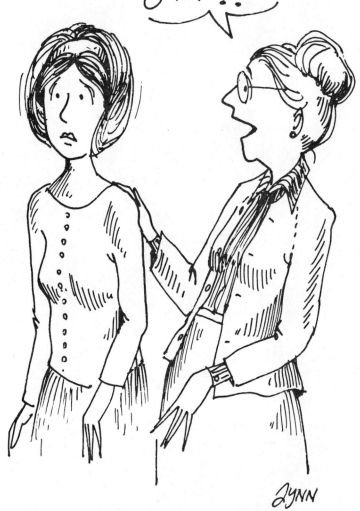

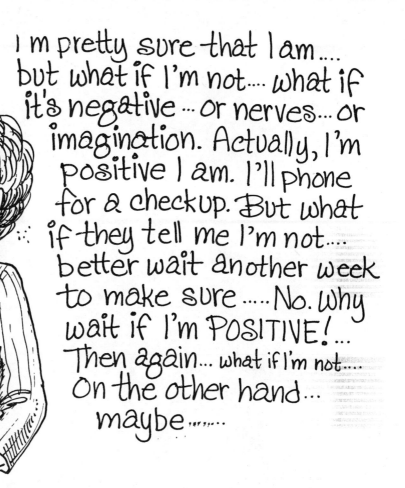

I'm pretty sure that I am.... but what if I'm not.... what if it's negative... or nerves... or imagination. Actually, I'm positive I am. I'll phone for a checkup. But what if they tell me I'm not.... better wait another week to make sure.....No. Why wait if I'm POSITIVE!... Then again... what if I'm not.... On the other hand... maybe........

Lynn

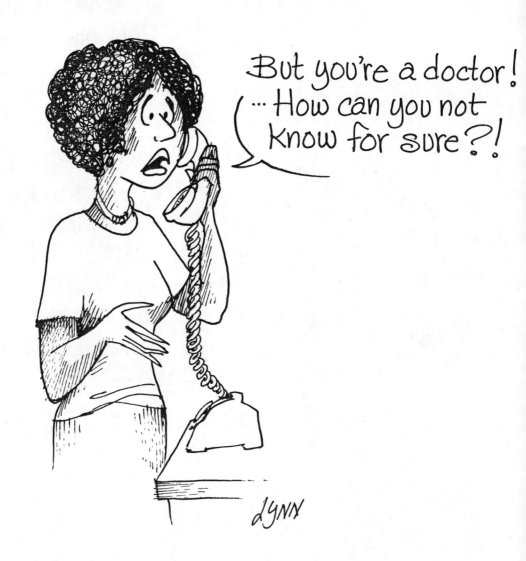

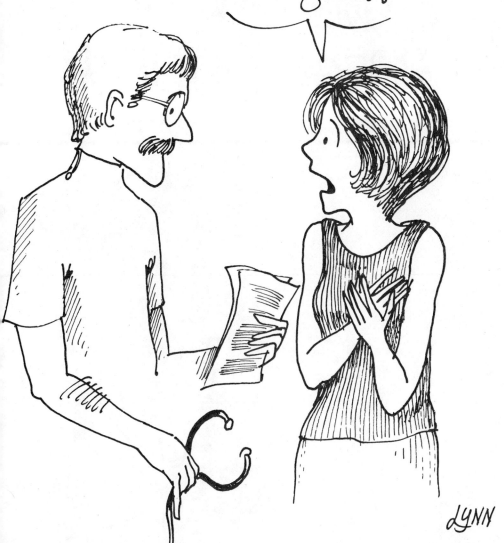

19

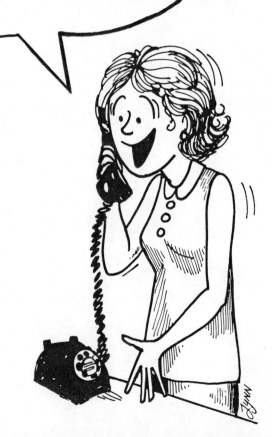

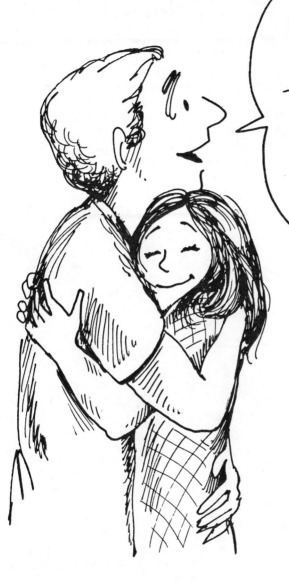

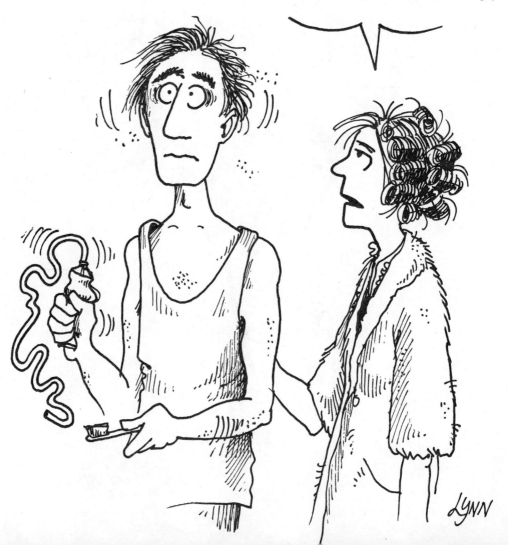

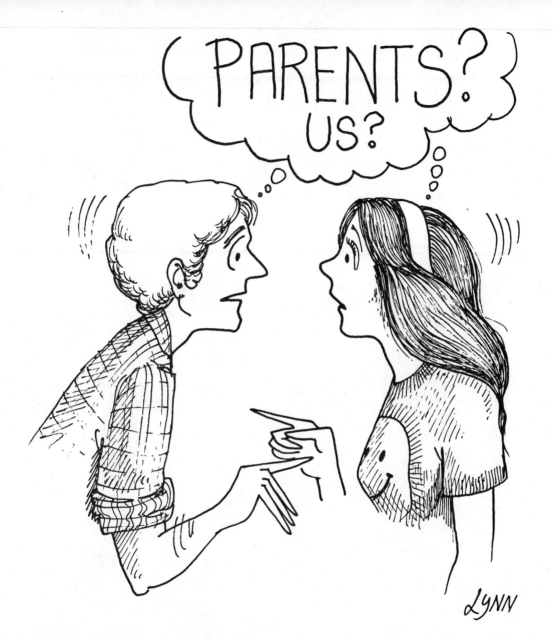

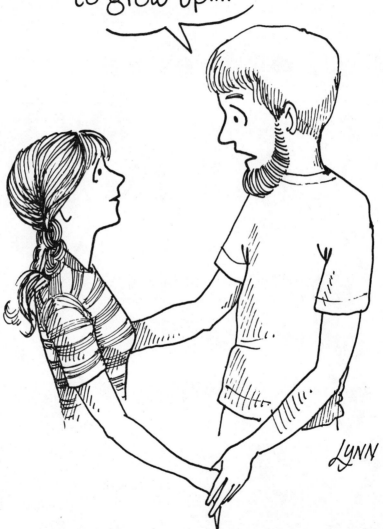

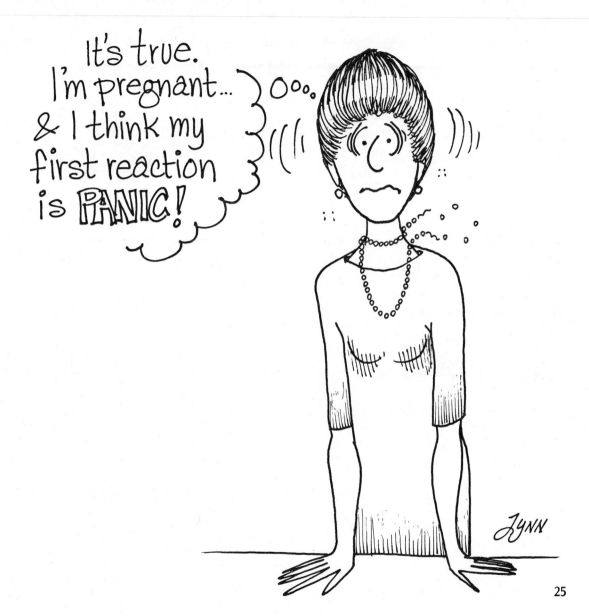

25

26

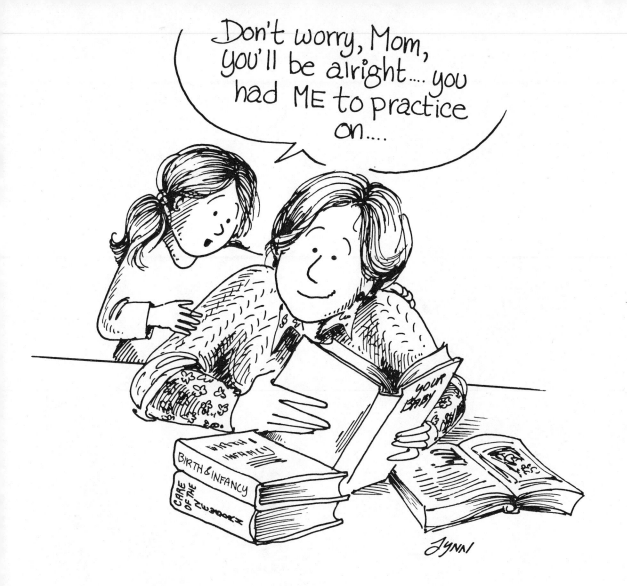

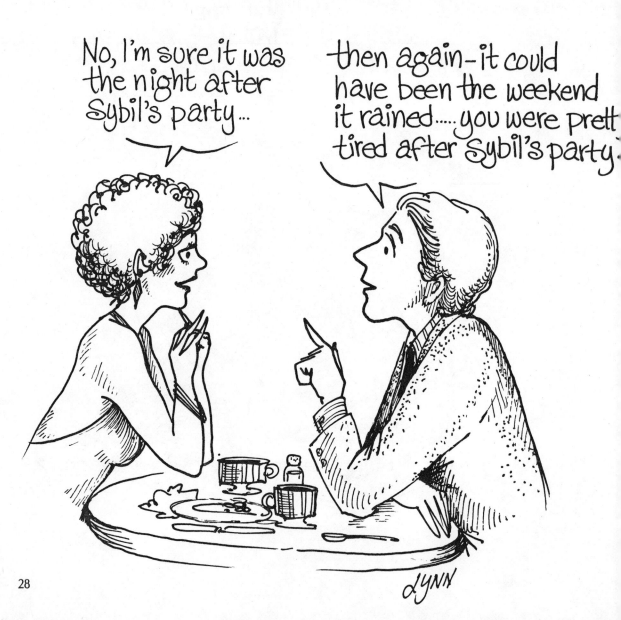

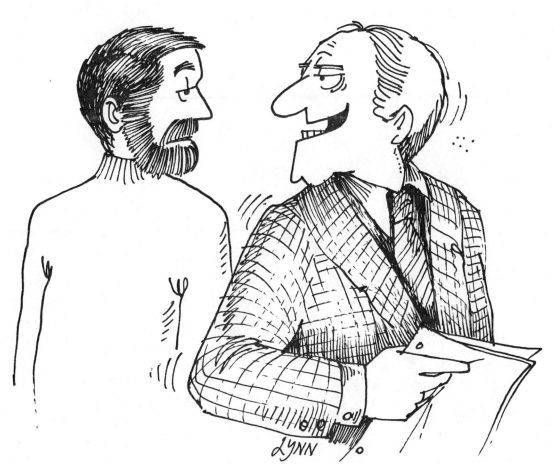

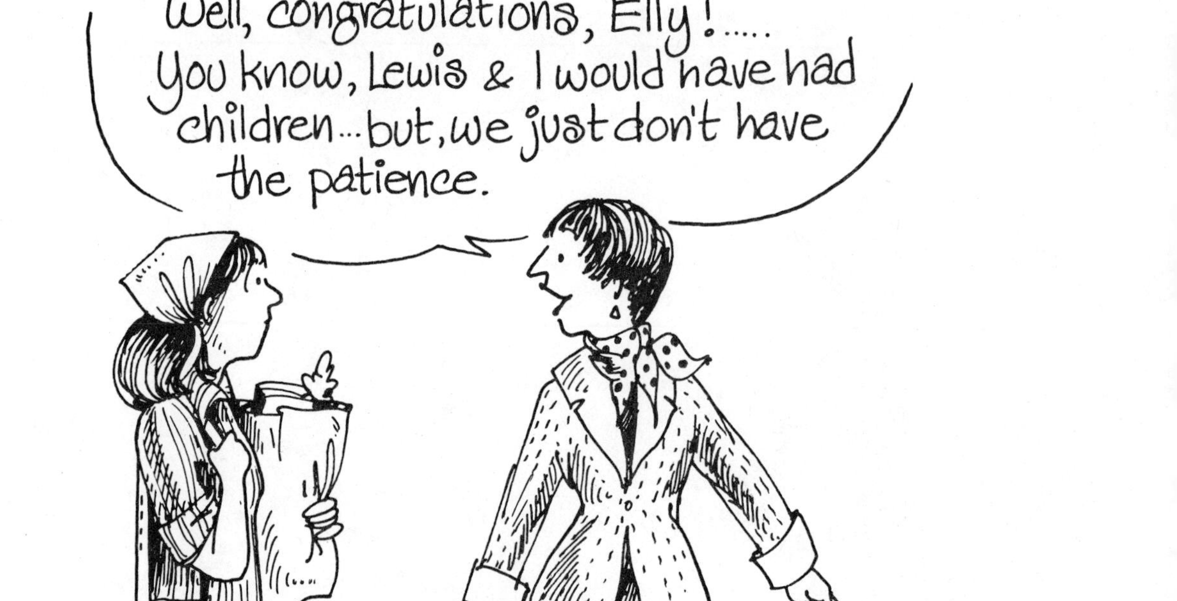
Well, congratulations, Elly!..... You know, Lewis & I would have had children...but, we just don't have the patience.
LYNN

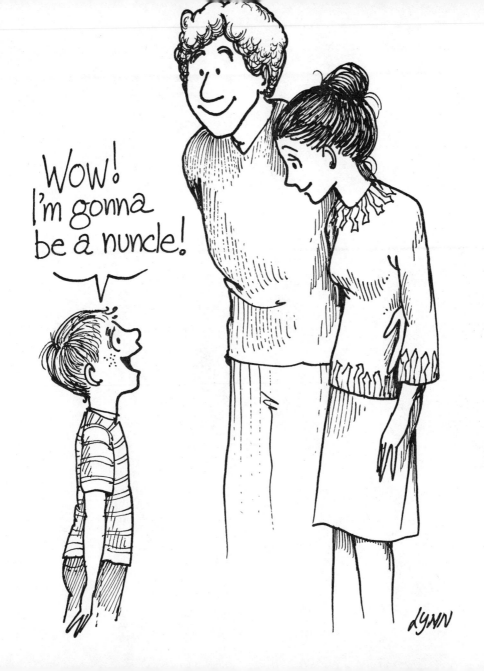

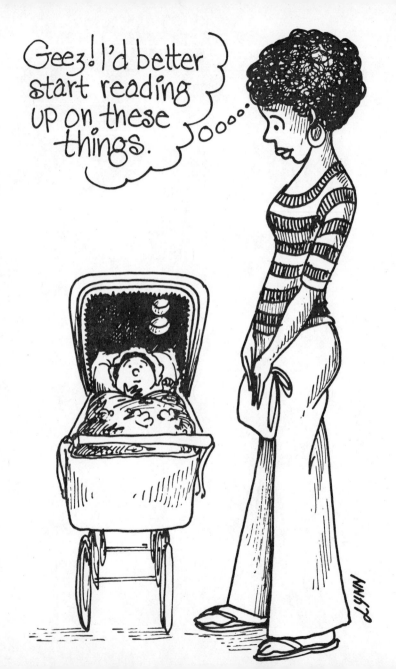

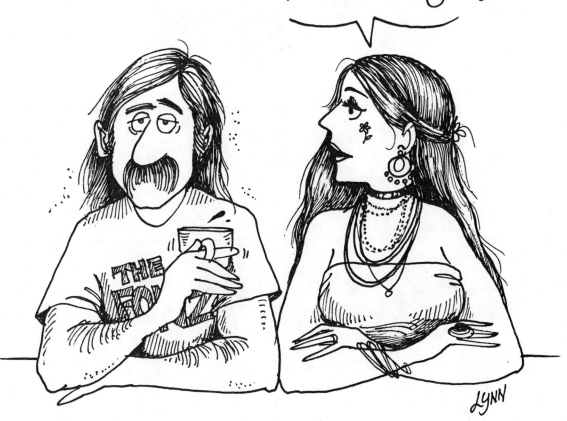

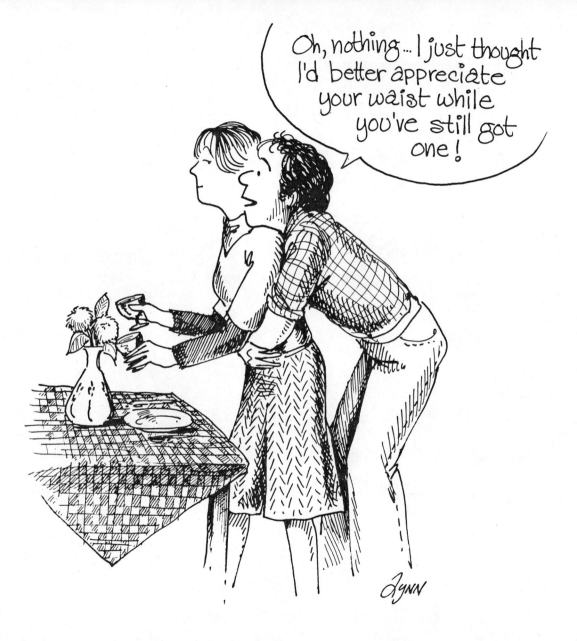

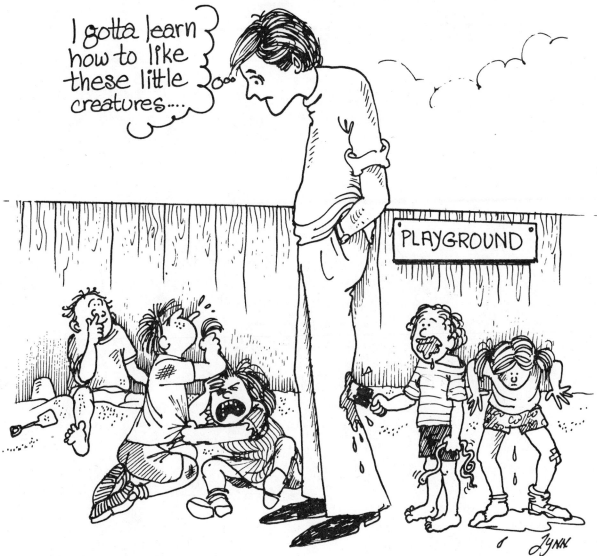

35

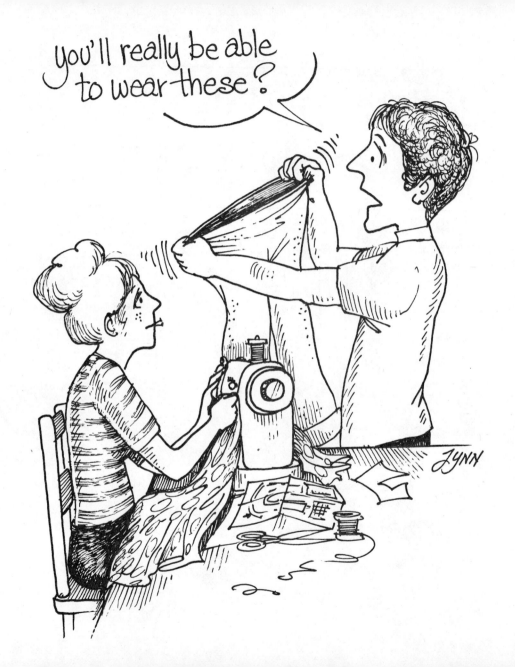

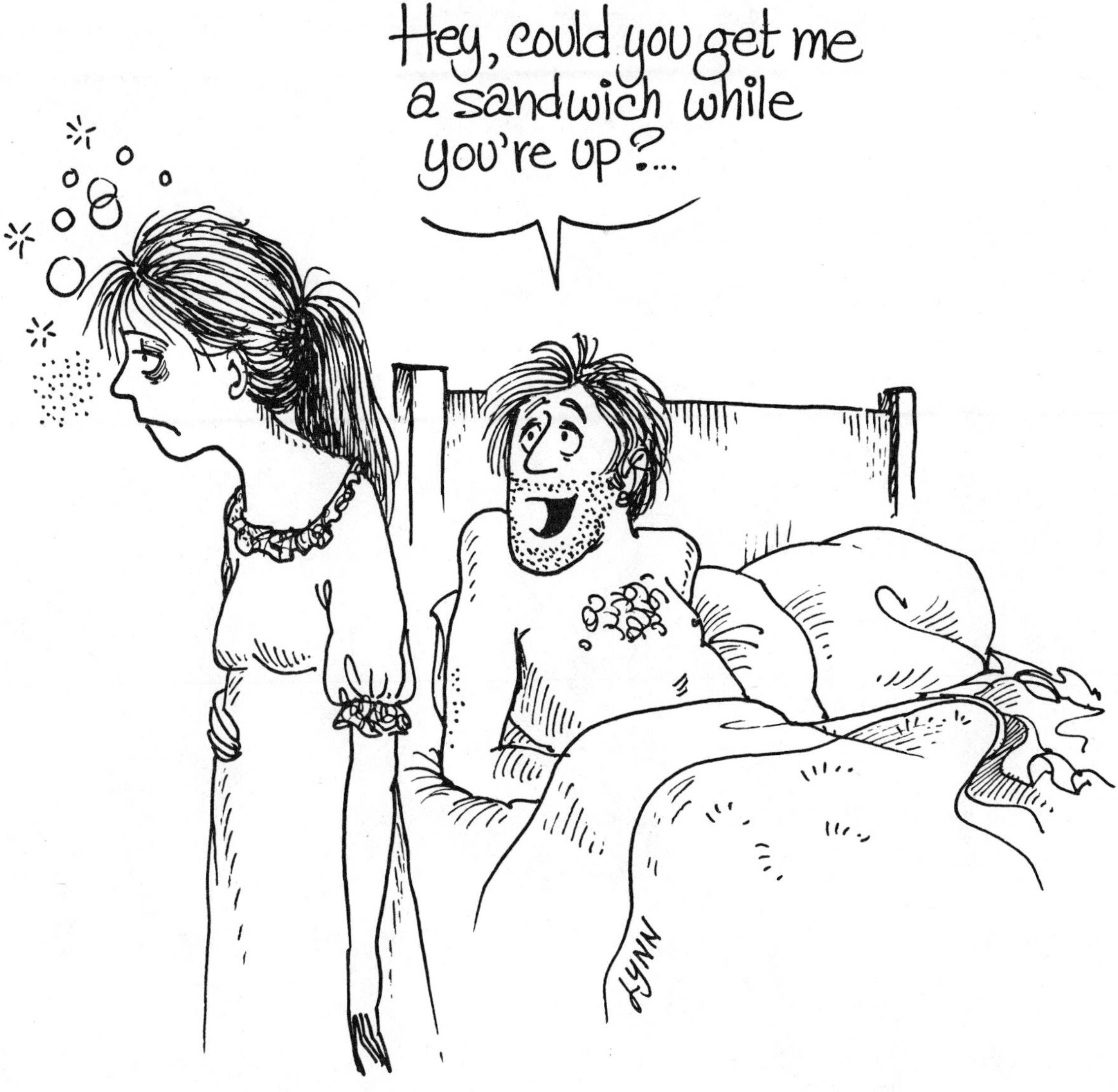
Hey, could you get me a sandwich while you're up?...
LYNN

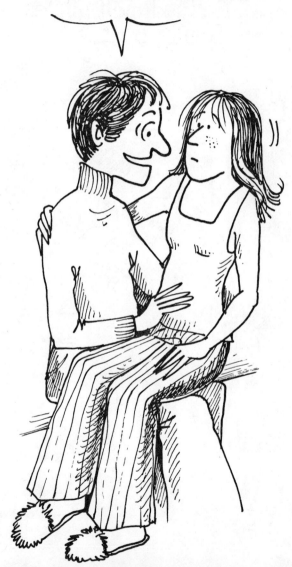

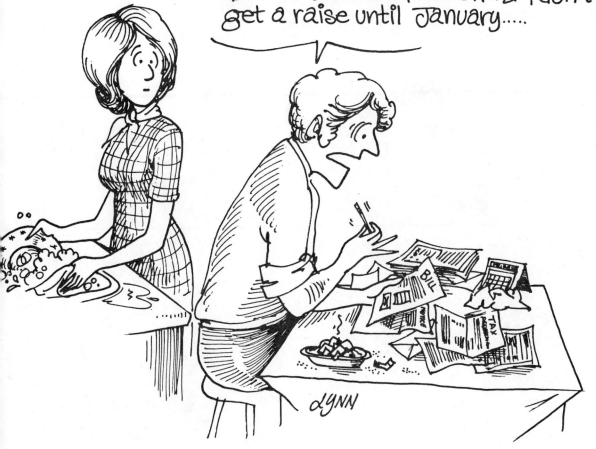

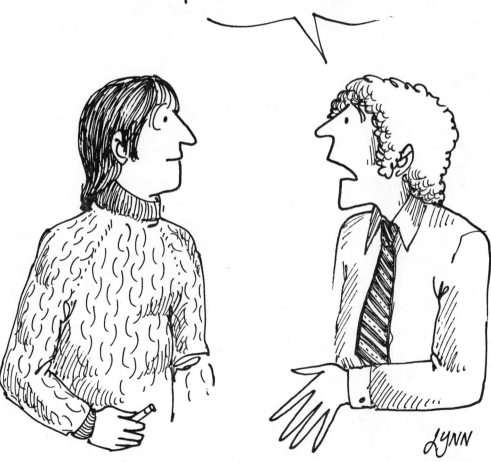

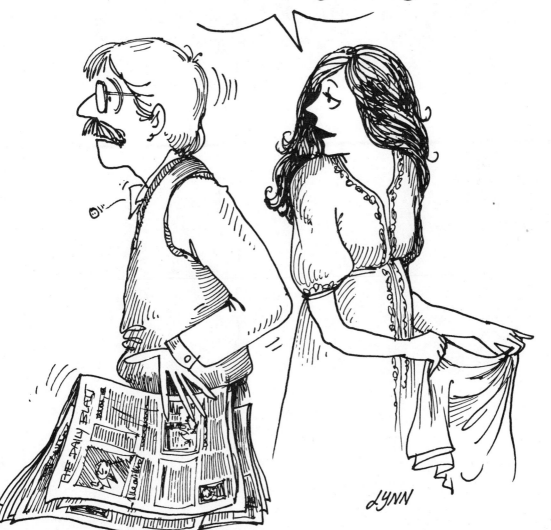

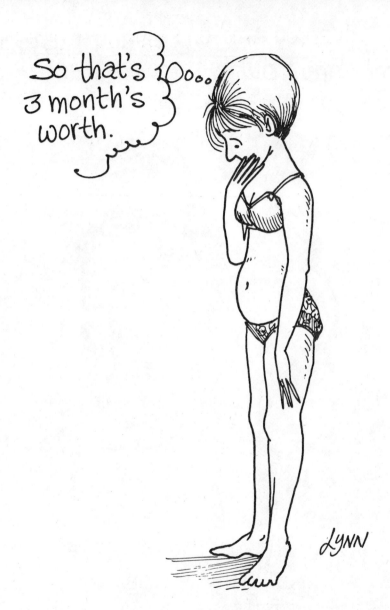

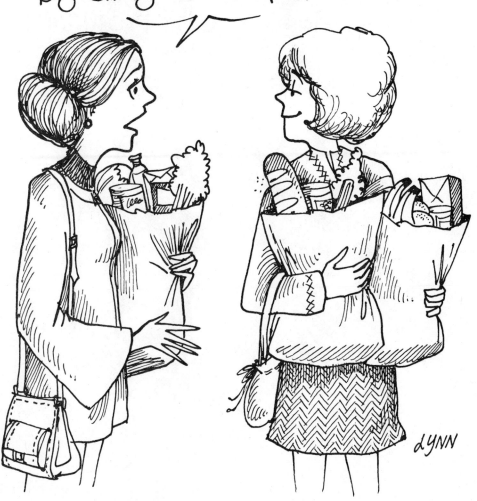

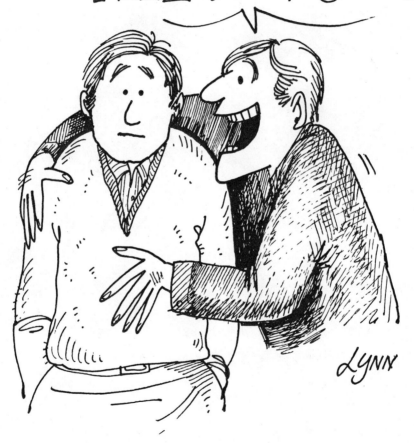

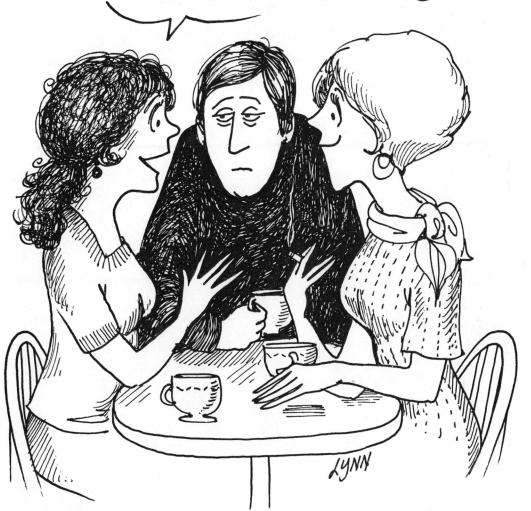

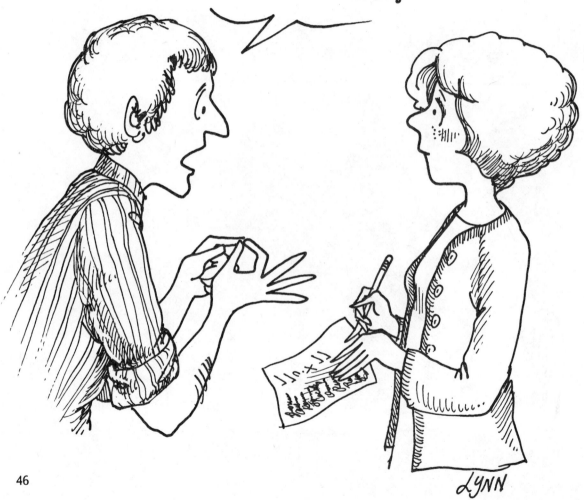

46

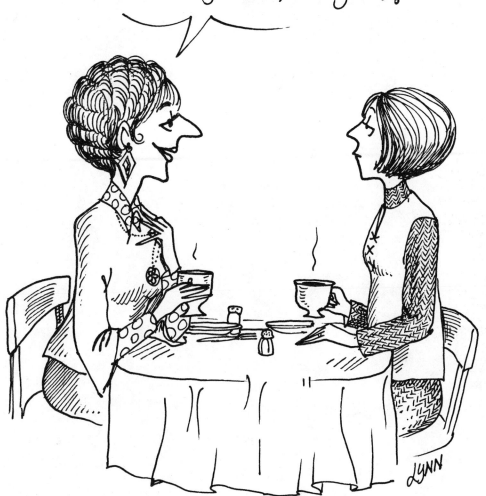

48

49

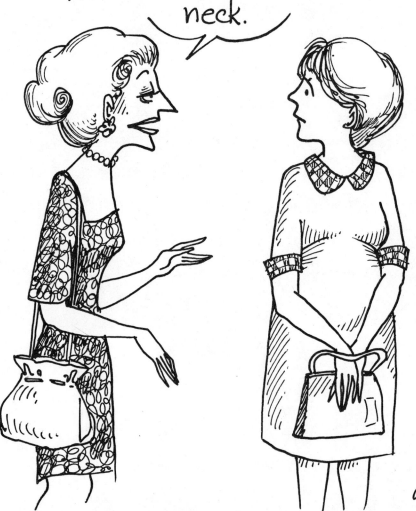

50

LYNN

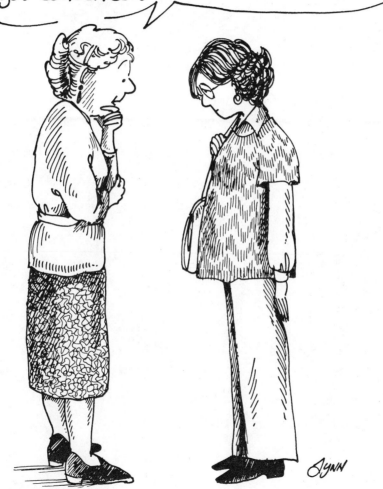

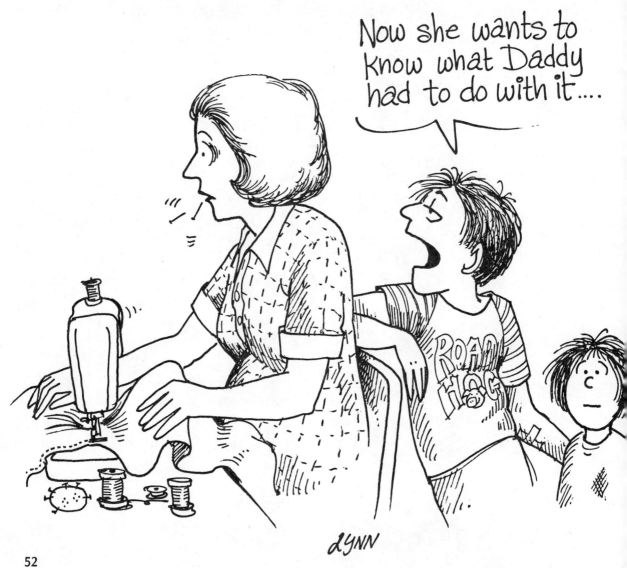

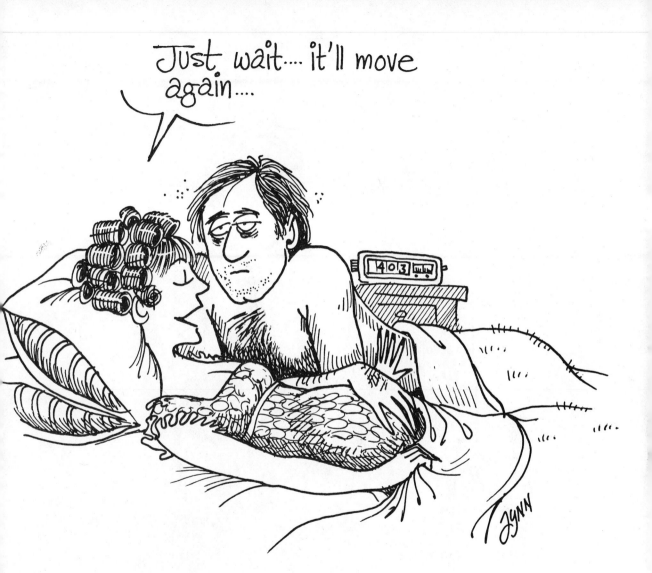

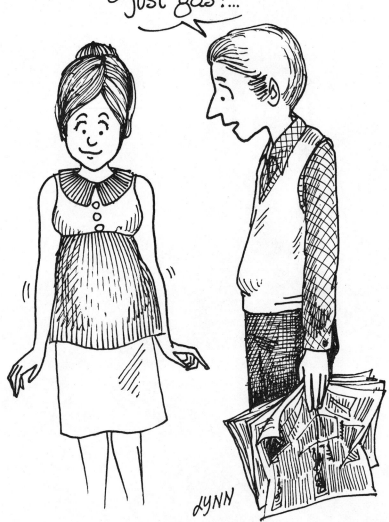

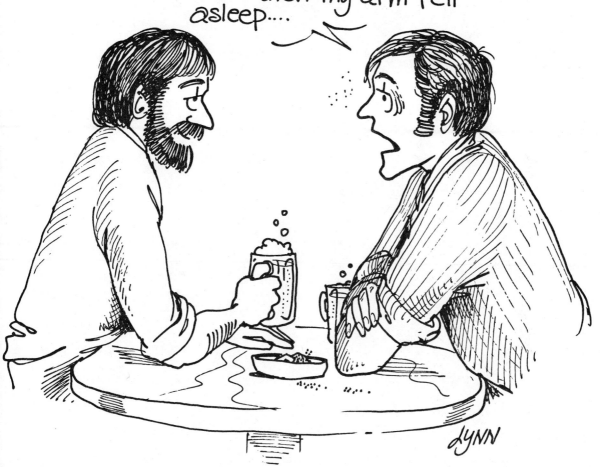

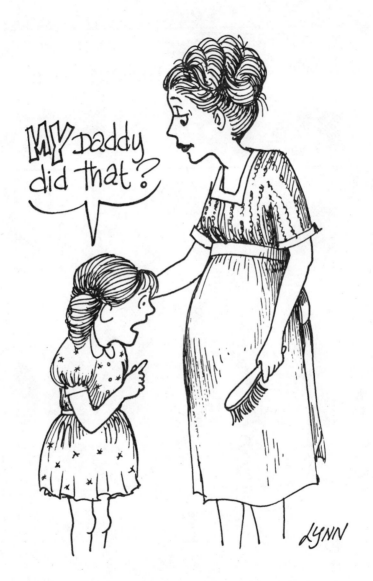

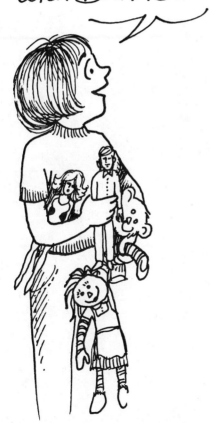

Mom, Ken's agreed to go to prenatal classes with Barbie....

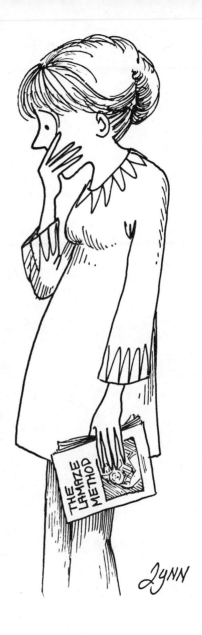

Lynn

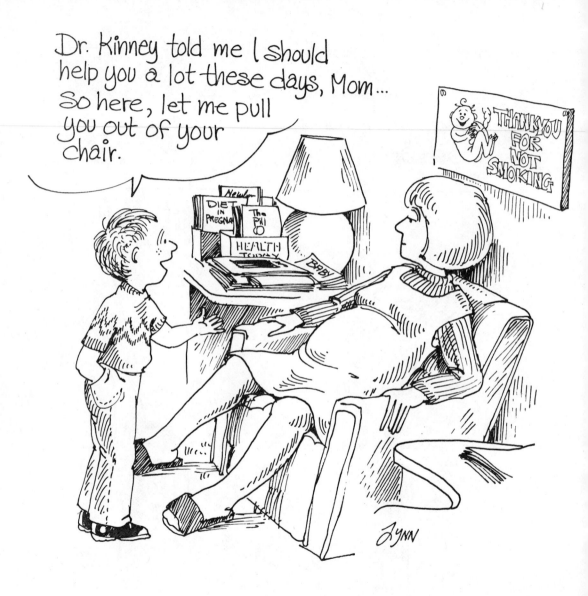

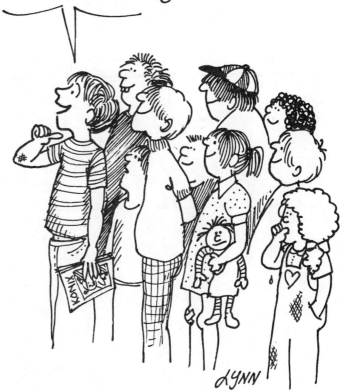
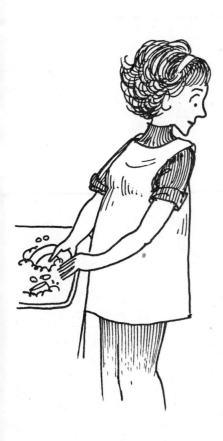

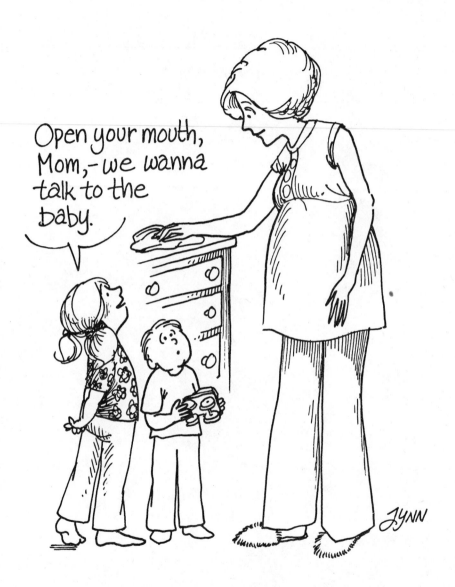

61

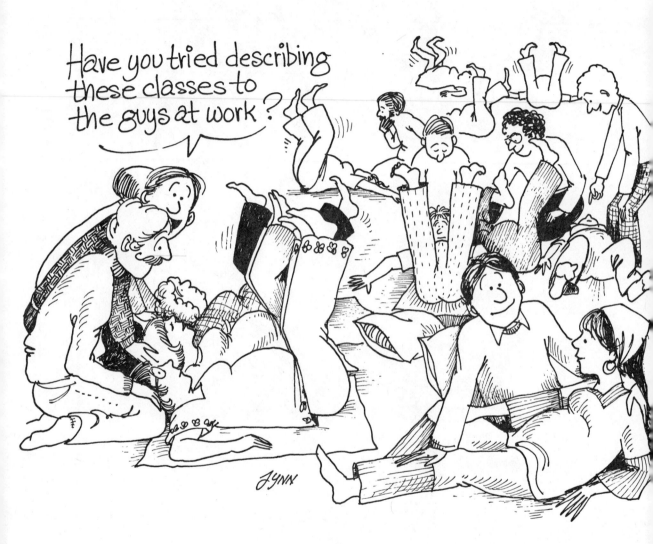

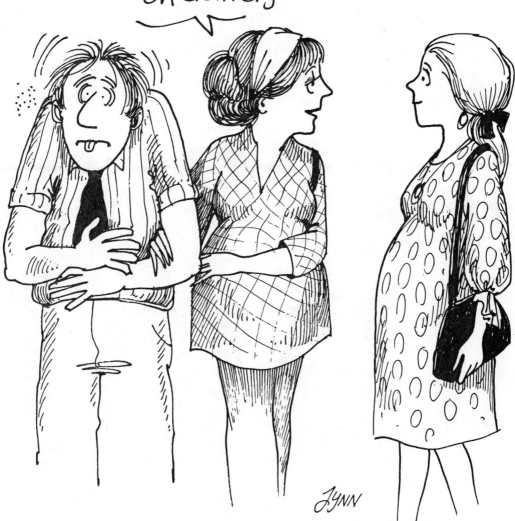

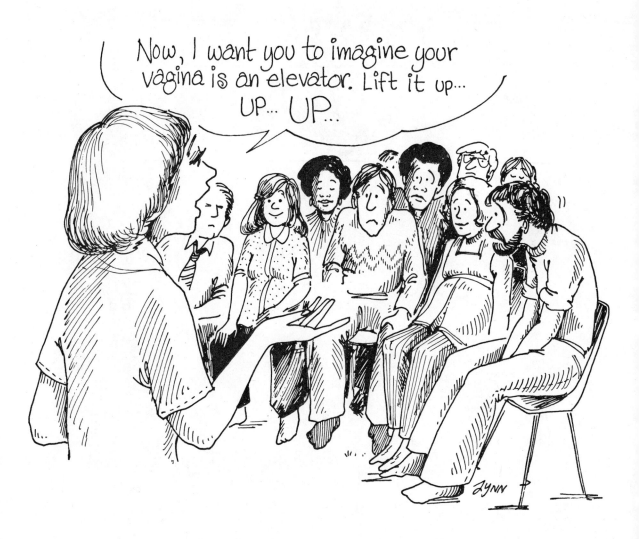

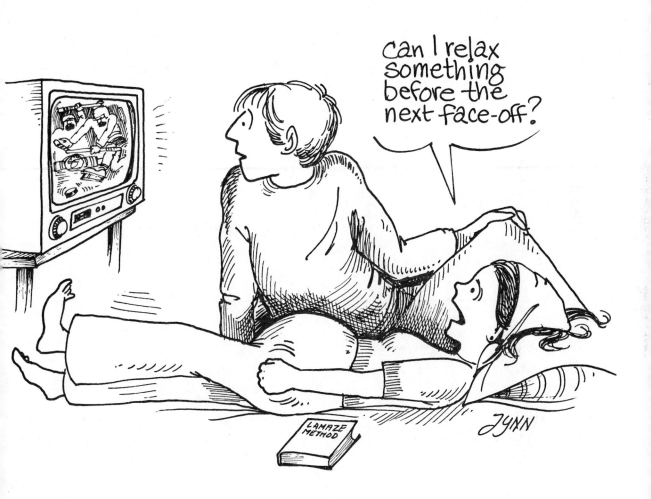

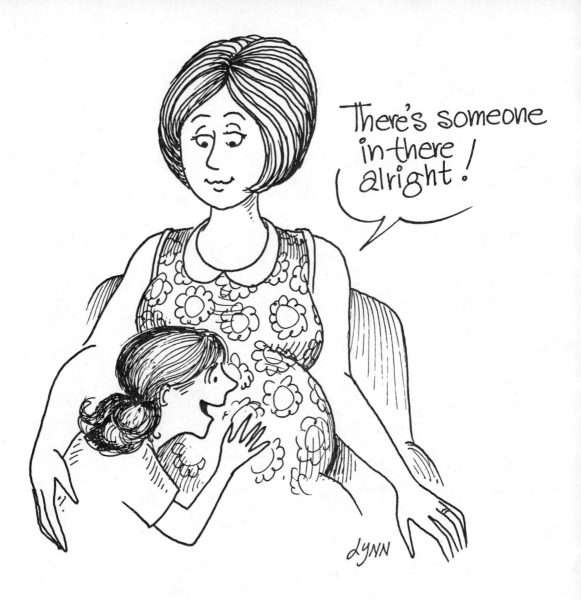

Mother's coming to give you the benefit of her experience....

LYNN

While you're waddling around town – could you pick me up a copy of the evening edition?

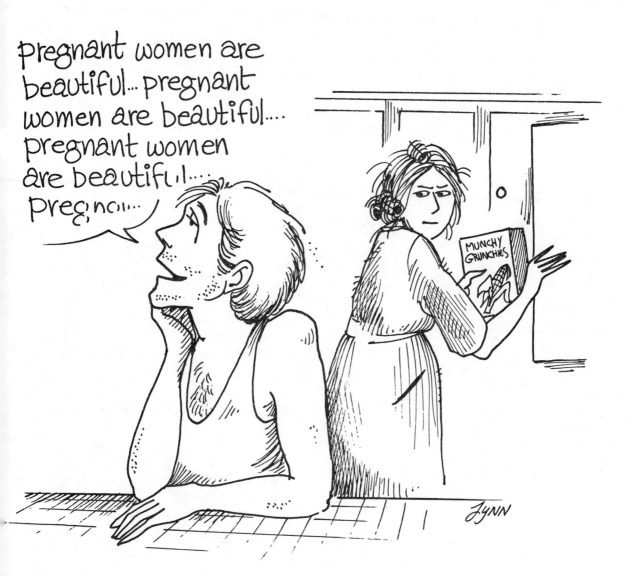

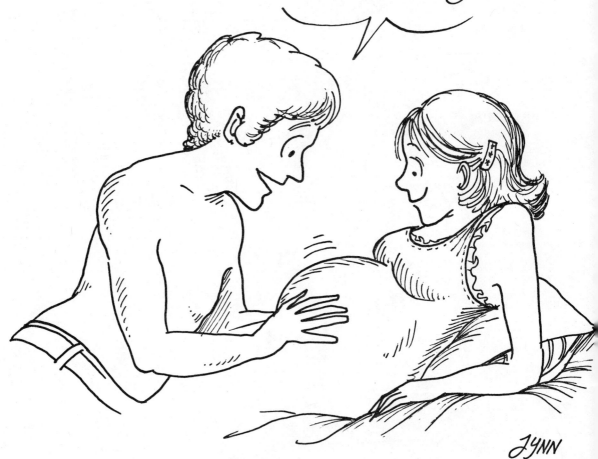

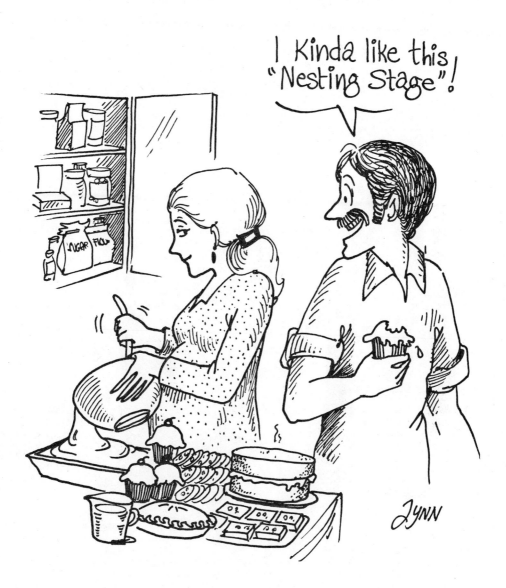

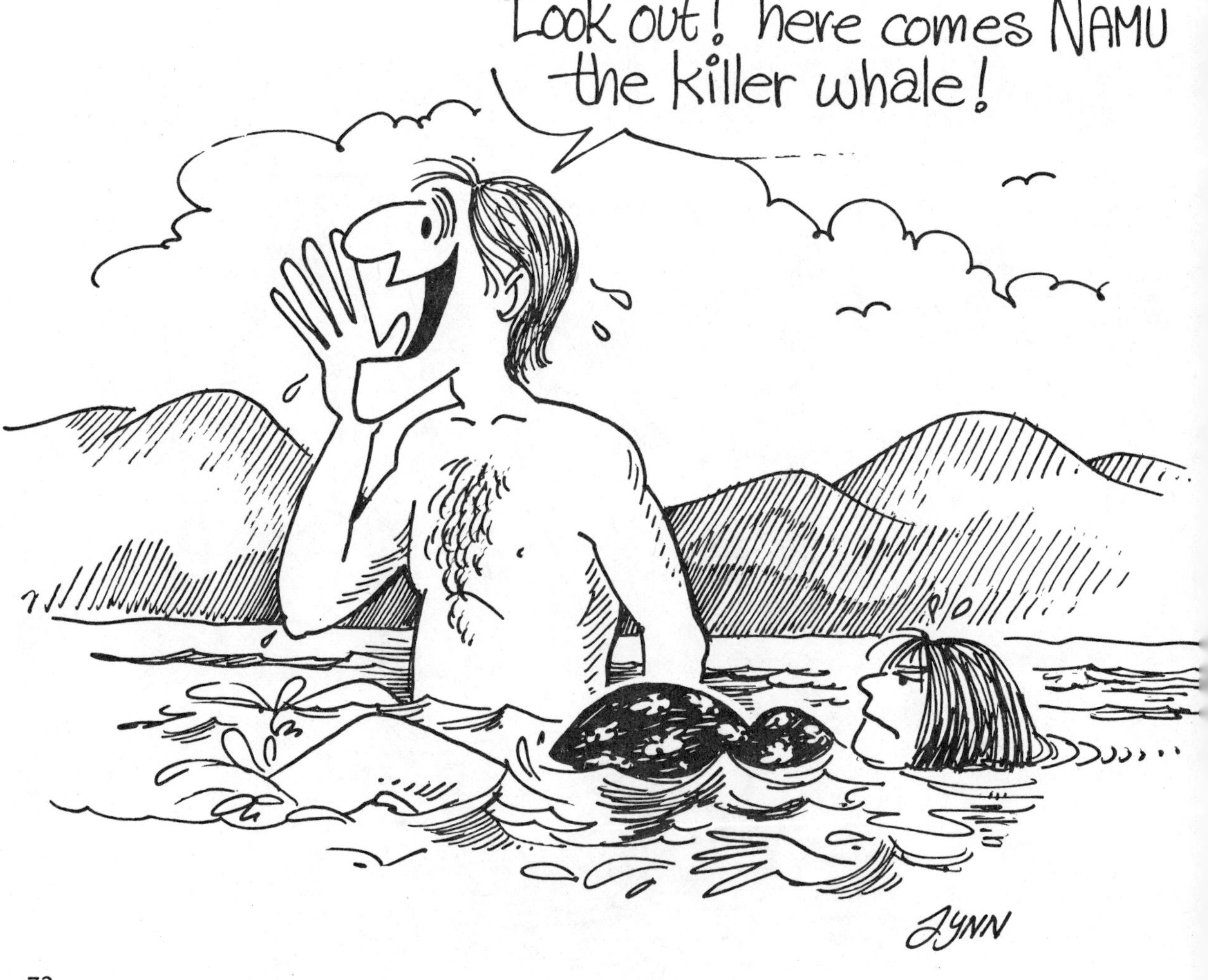

Look out! here comes NAMU the killer whale!
LYNN

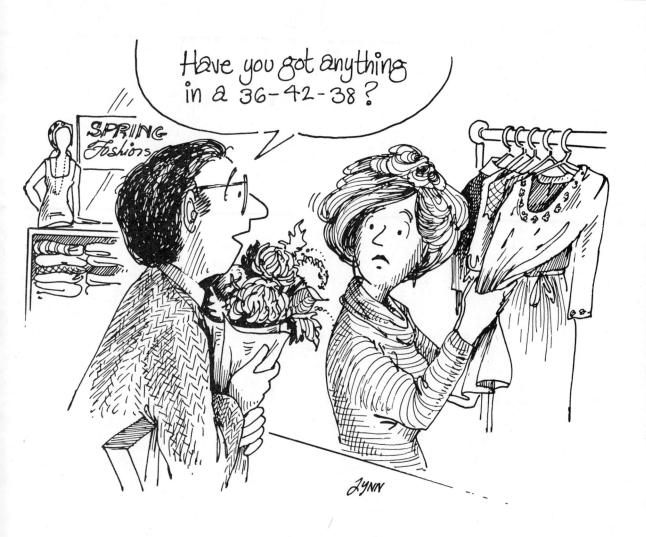

No matter how I lie, I'm uncomfortable.... I think I'm going to have to learn how to sleep standing up.

ZZZZZ

LYNN

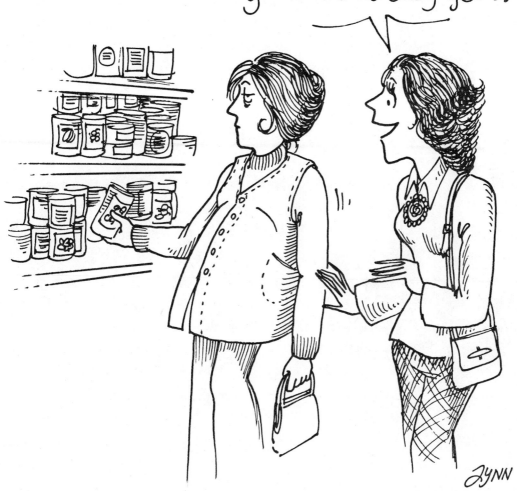

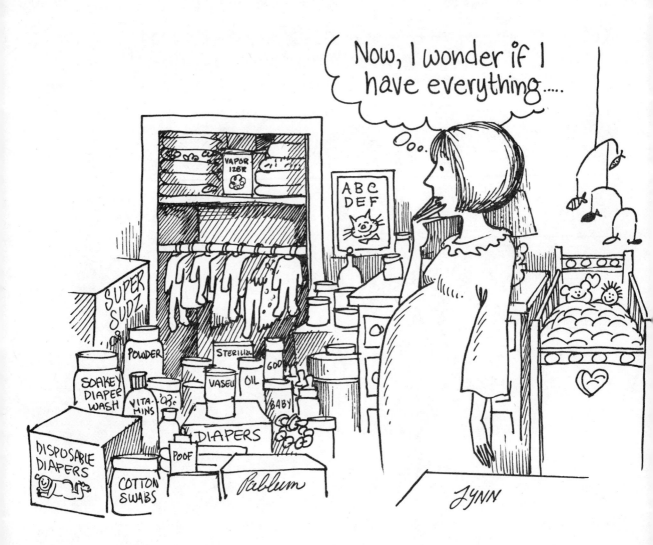

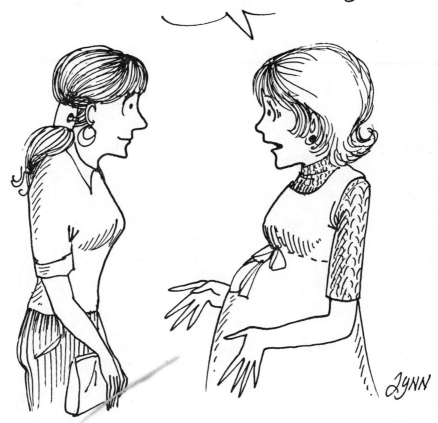

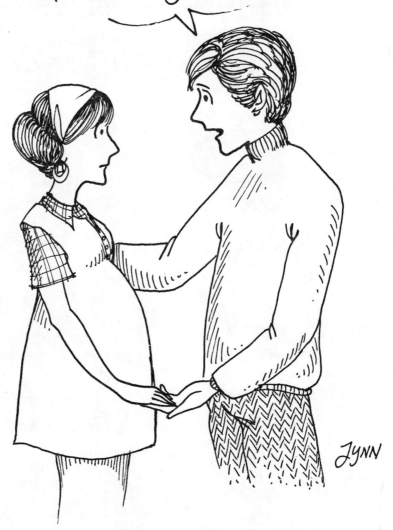

79

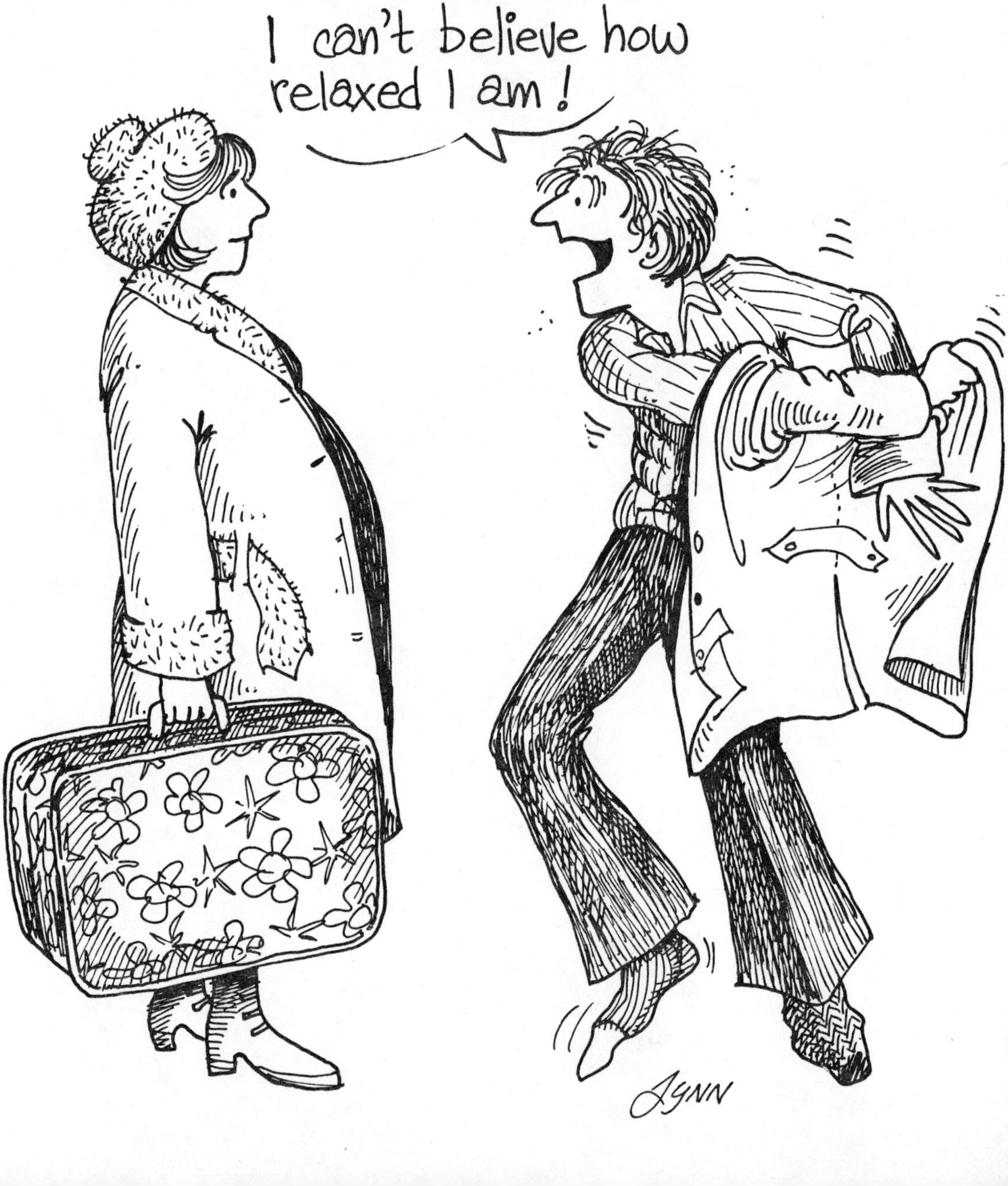
I can't believe how relaxed I am!
LYNN

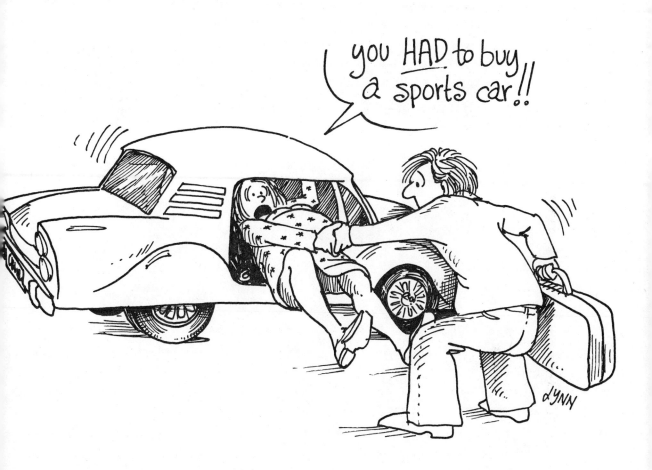

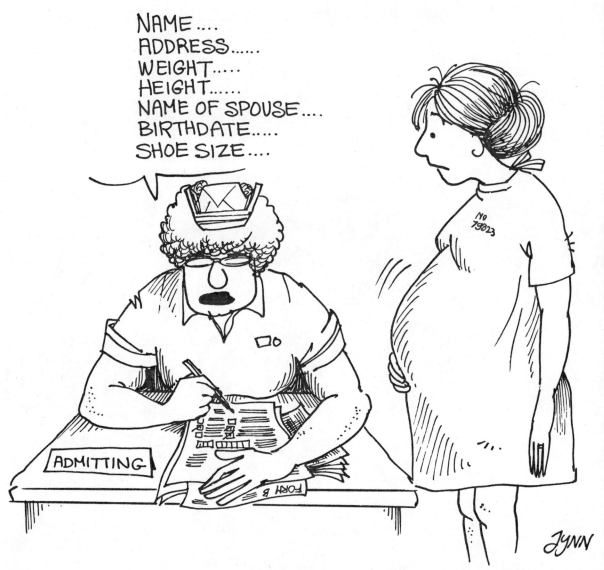

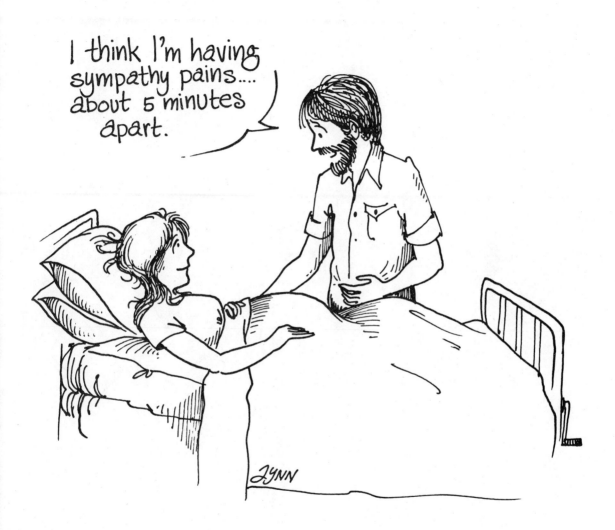

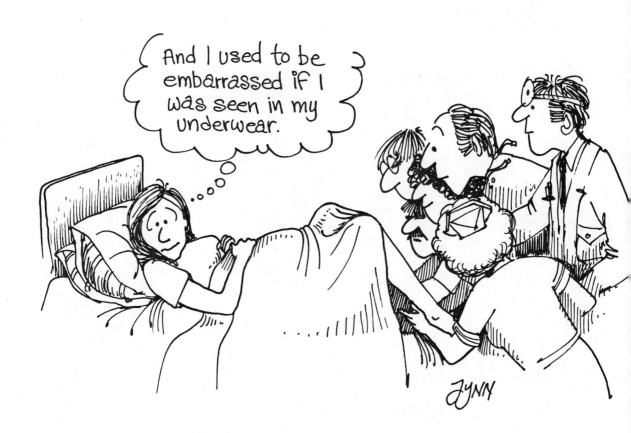

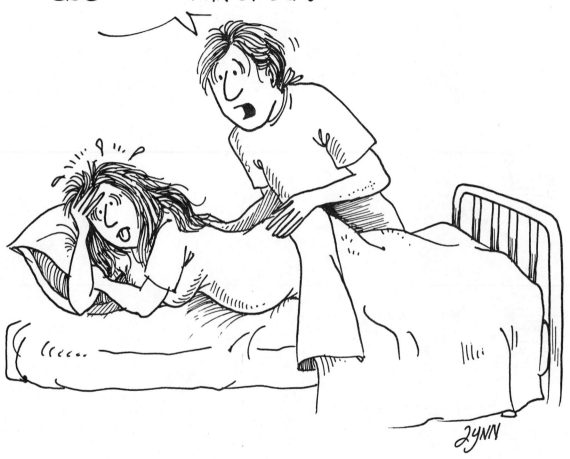

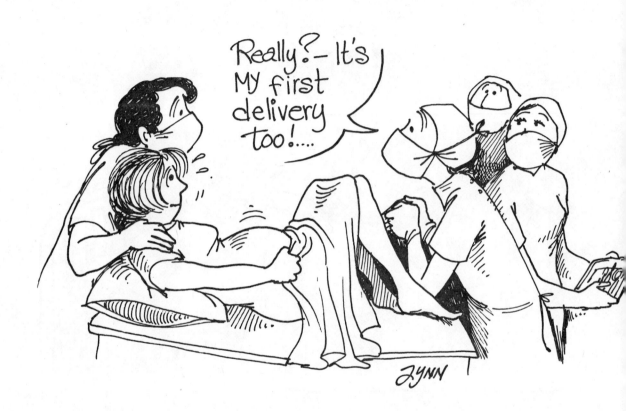

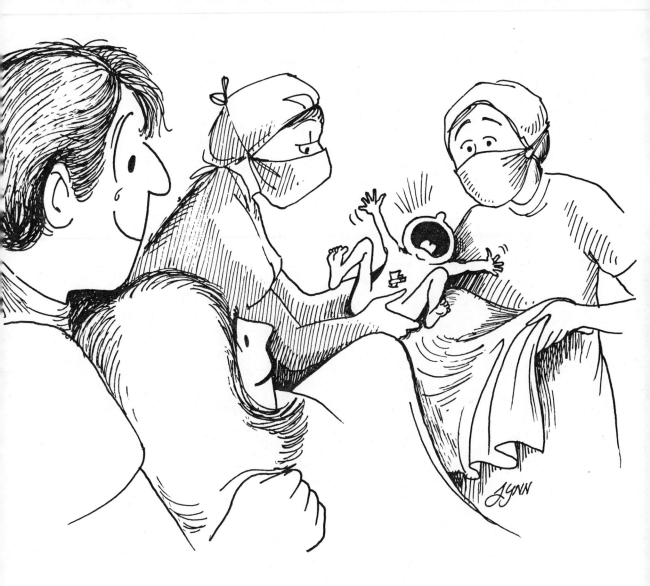

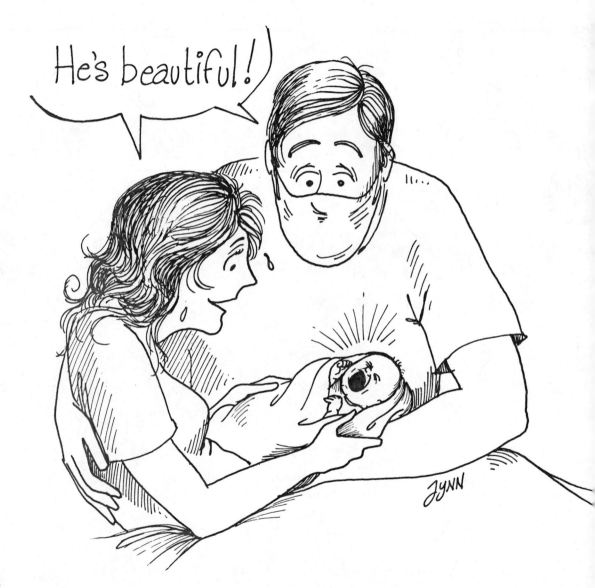

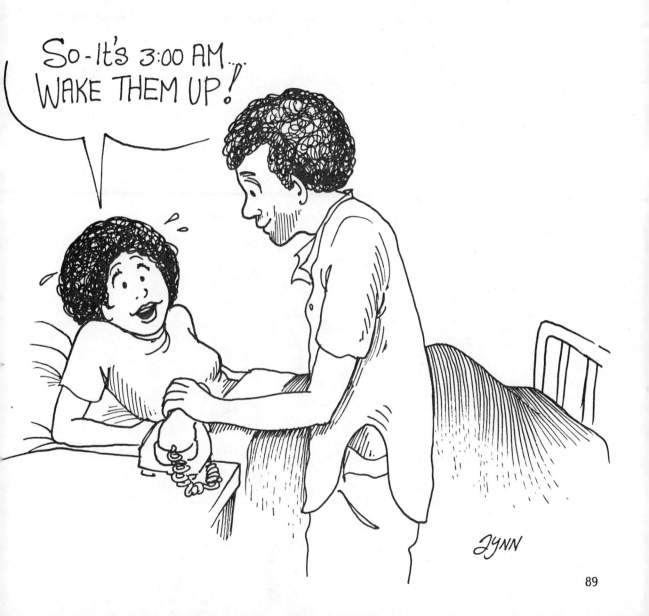

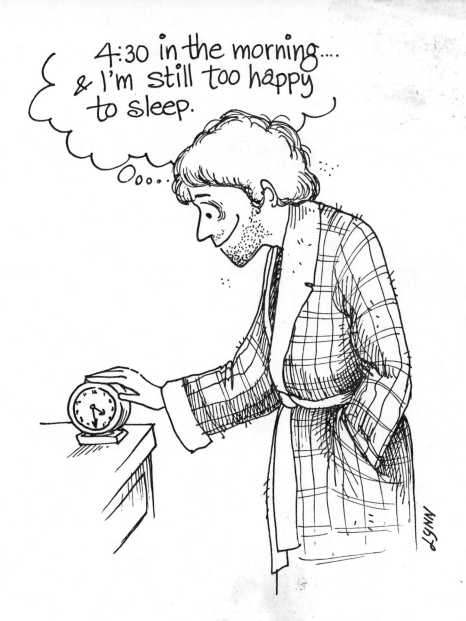

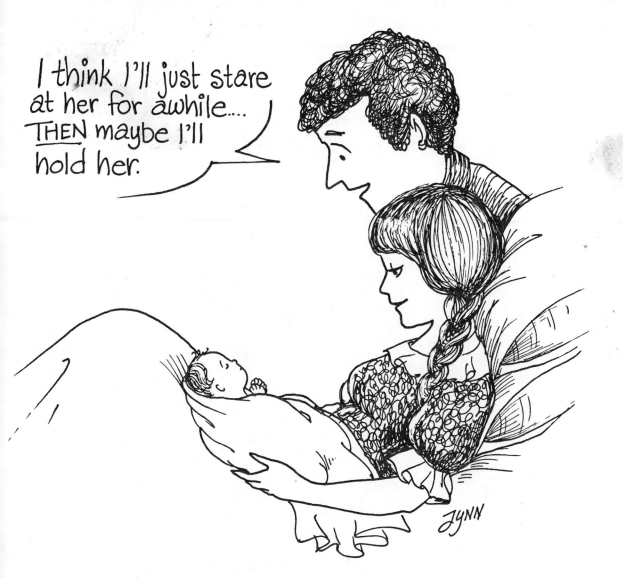

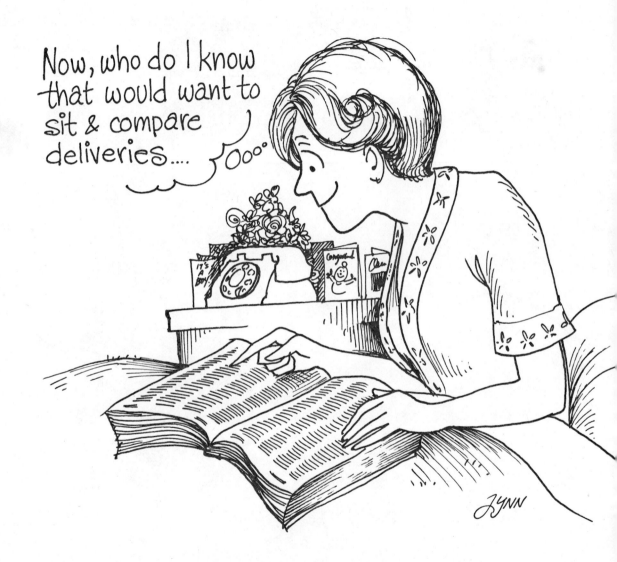

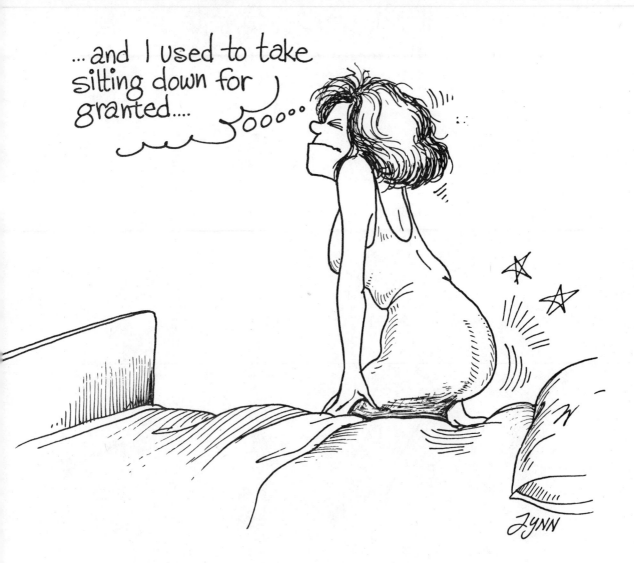

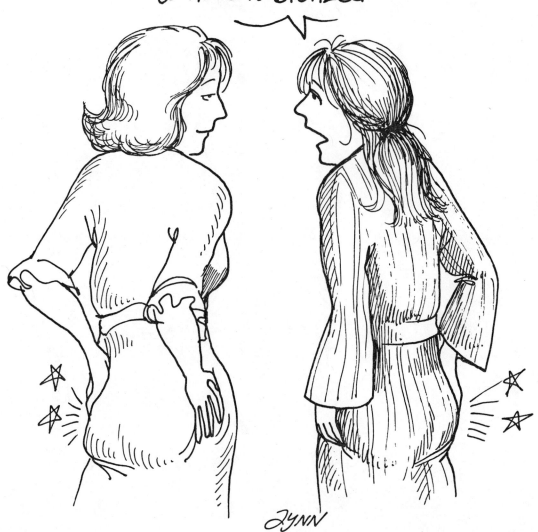

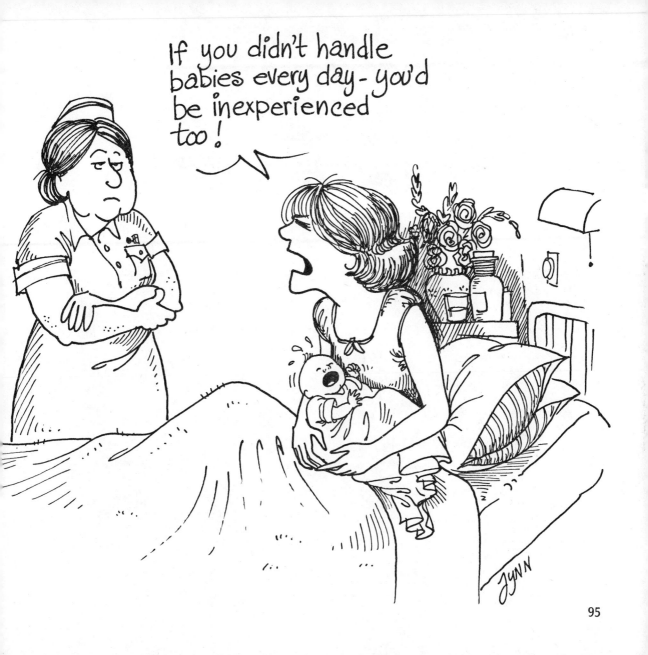

95

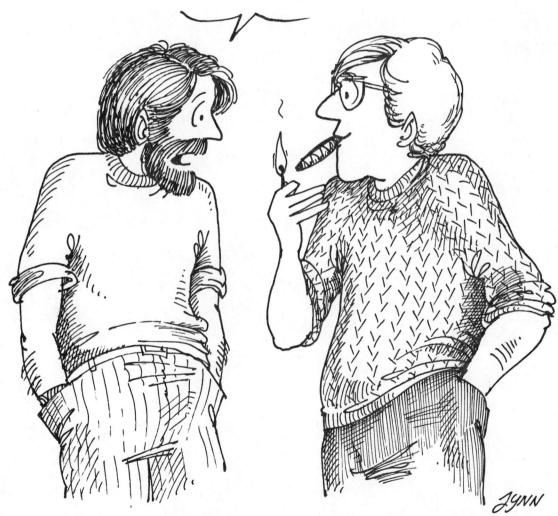

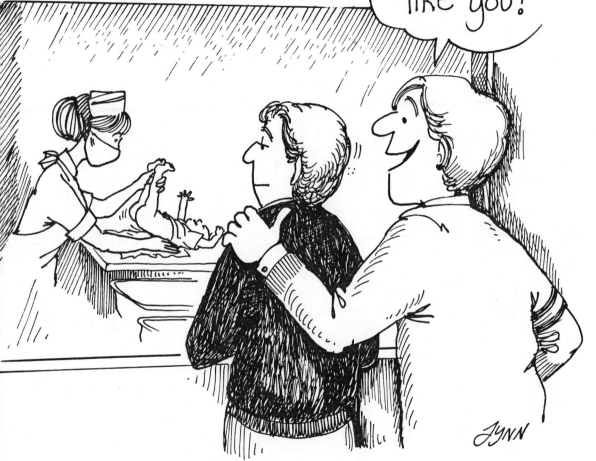

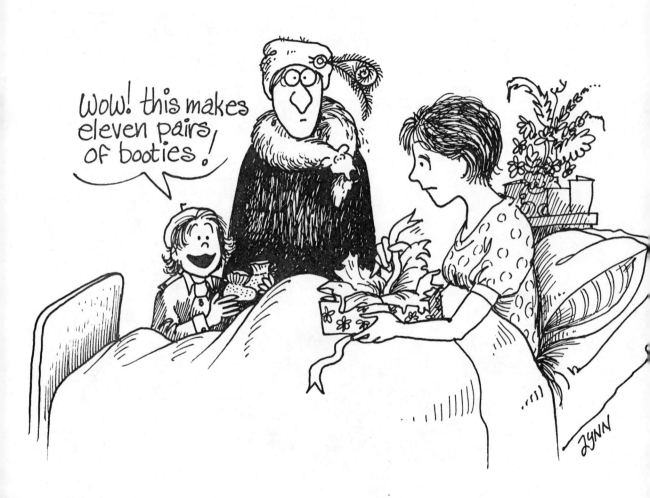

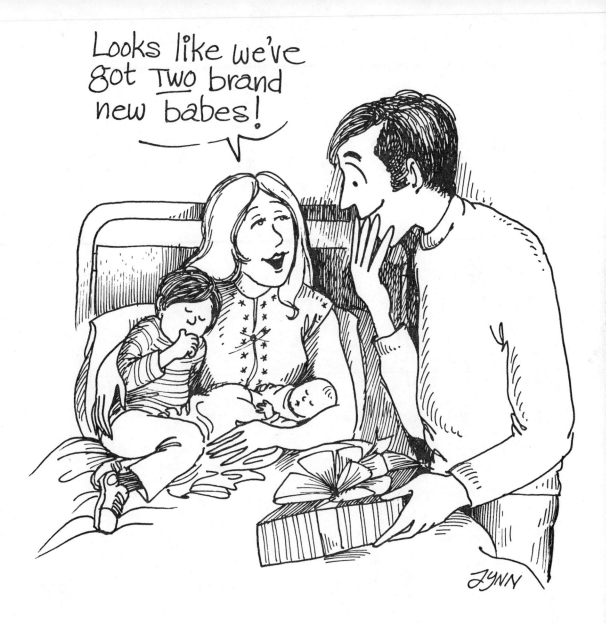

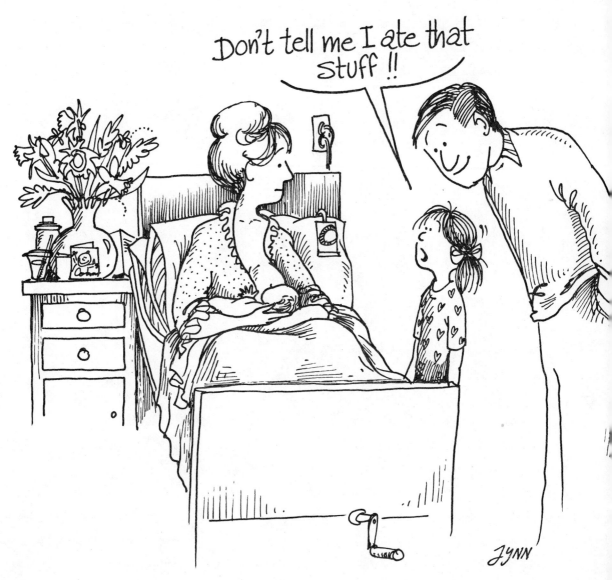

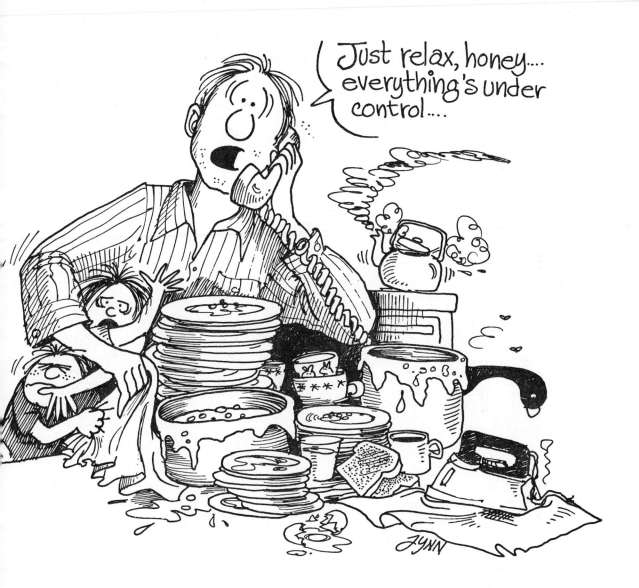

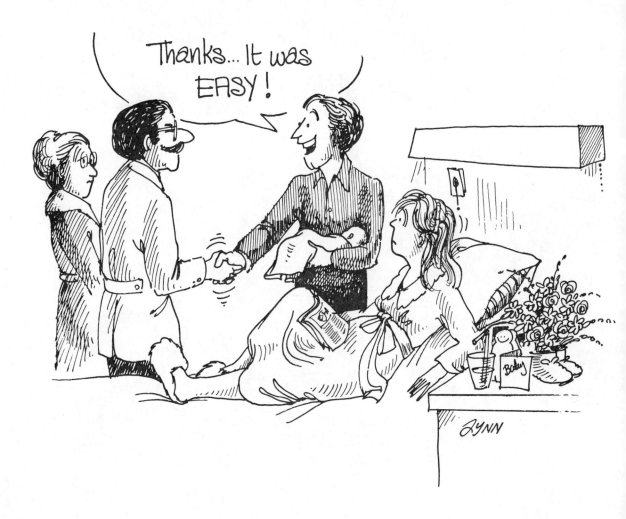

102

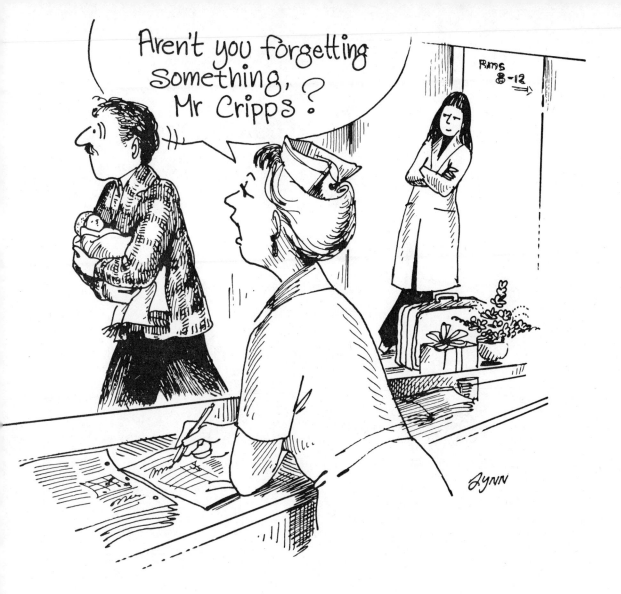

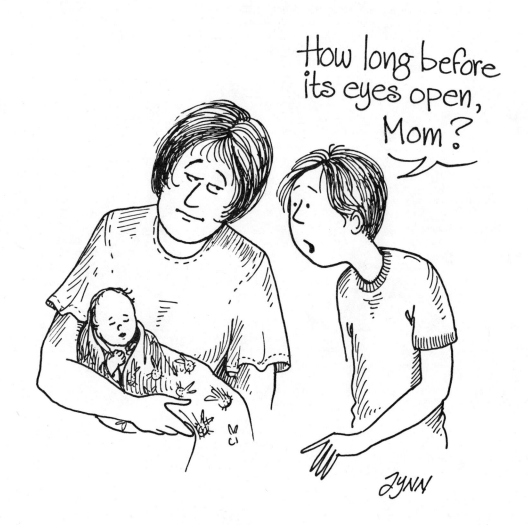

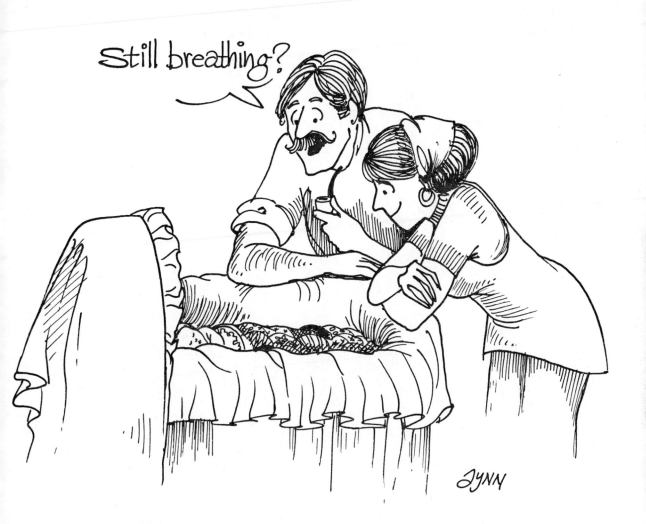

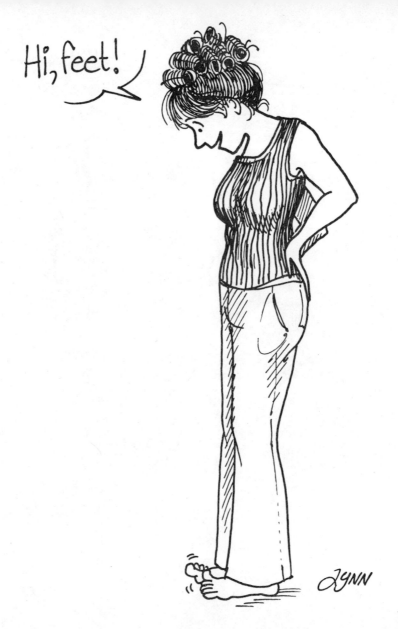

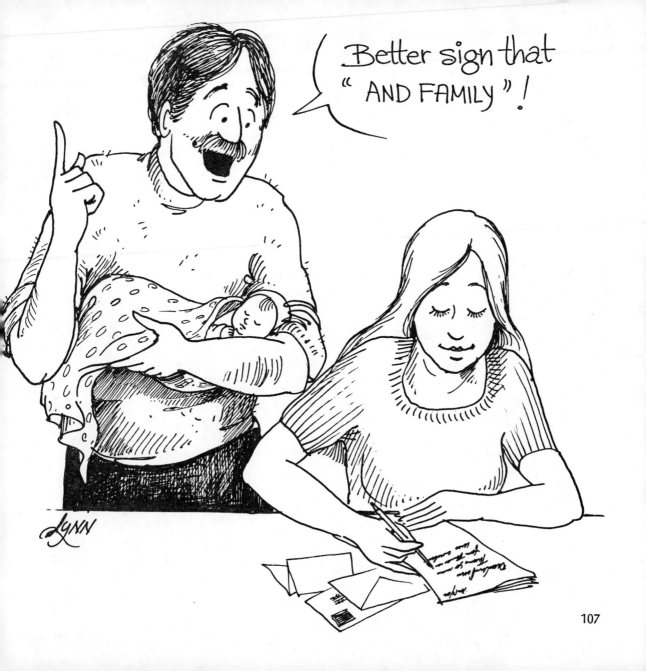

107

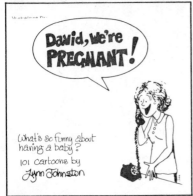
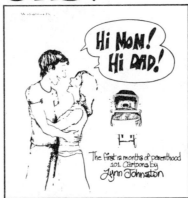
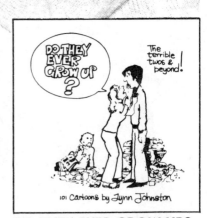

FREE STUFF BOOKS

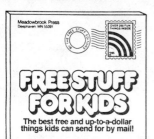

FREE STUFF FOR KIDS
Over 250 of the best free and up-to-a-dollar things kids can get by mail:
- coins & stamps
- bumper stickers & decals
- posters & maps

$3.75 ppd.

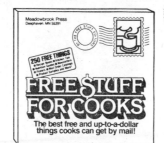

FREE STUFF FOR COOKS
Over 250 of the best free and up-to-a-dollar booklets and samples cooks can get by mail:
- cookbooks & recipe cards
- money-saving shopping guides
- seeds & spices

$3.75 ppd.

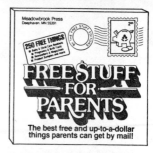

FREE STUFF FOR PARENTS
Over 250 of the best free and up-to-a-dollar booklets and samples parents can get by mail:
- sample teethers
- booklets on pregnancy & childbirth
- sample newsletters

$3.75 ppd.

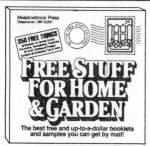

FREE STUFF FOR HOME & GARDEN
Over 350 of the best free and up-to-a-dollar booklets and samples homeowners and gardeners can get by mail:
- booklets on home improvement & energy
- plans for do-it-yourself projects

$3.75 ppd.

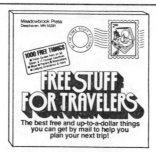

FREE STUFF FOR TRAVELERS
Over 1,000 of the best free and up-to-a-dollar publications and products travelers can get by mail:
- guidebooks to cities, states & foreign countries
- pamphlets on attractions, festivals & parks
- posters, calendars & maps

$3.75 ppd.

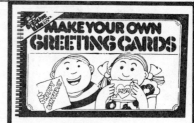

MAKE YOUR OWN GREETING CARDS
Now it's easy and fun to make your own greeting cards with stencils!
- birthday cards, invitations, get-well notes
- cards for Christmas, Halloween, Valentine's, Mother's and Father's Day (and more)
- postcards, stationery and special messages!

$5.75 ppd.

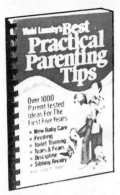
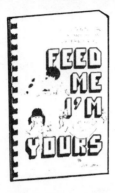
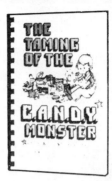
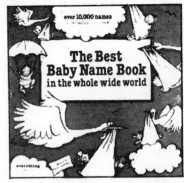